Speak Up

Assertive Communication for Healthy Boundaries

Table of Contents

Chapter 1. Introduction

Welcome to this Special Report: "Speak Up: Assertive Communication for Healthy Boundaries!" This is not just another report, but your key to unlocking a harmonious life balance and nurturing profound relationships in every sphere of life! Culled from expert insights and practical examples, this eye-opening report is tailored to teach you the magic of assertiveness and the art of setting healthy boundaries with grace and tact. It's your turn to gear up, embrace your true potential and power. Start your transformational journey today! Whether you are a novice or a seasoned communicator, this guide is made for you. Let's dive into the world of assertive communication together! Come, join the chorus of many who've already benefitted and are marching towards a self-assured future with stronger, healthier boundaries!

Chapter 2. The Foundation of Assertive Communication

Assertive communication is firmly rooted in a deep understanding of oneself coupled with empathy towards others. It represents a fundamental shift from reactive to proactive communication, anchored on the twin pedestals of self-respect and respect for others' perspectives.

2.1. Understanding Assertiveness

The term "assertiveness" is often misunderstood as being aggressive or domineering. However, it is far from such a definition. Assertiveness involves expressing oneself effectively and standing up for one's point of view, without being abrasive or disregarding others' rights.

Assertiveness is the assurance that you can get your point across respectfully, without offending or being offensive. It involves open, straightforward expressions and behaviours. When a person is assertive, they feel free to express their feelings, thoughts, desires, and reactions to others' beliefs or actions. Contrary to popular belief, being assertive does not mean one is unkind or disrespectful. Assertiveness embodies respect – for oneself and others.

2.2. The Importance of Self-Awareness

Fundamental to assertive communication is self-awareness. Being aware of one's feelings, thoughts, actions, and their impact on self and others is a prerequisite to effective assertive communication. Self-awareness drives self-control and aids in objective decision-making. Furthermore, it promotes empathy by enabling us to perceive others more realistically, and not simply through our own subjective lenses.

Become consciously aware of your thoughts and emotions. This cognizance helps articulate your needs and wants more clearly. Remember, understanding your emotions aids in managing them more effectively so they don't lead your responses impulsively.

2.3. Non-Assertive Versus Assertive Communication

To understand assertive communication, it is crucial to differentiate it from non-assertive or passive communication, and aggressive communication.

Non-assertive individuals avoid expressing their feelings or confrontations for fear of offending others. They place others' needs before their own, creating an imbalance of power. This can lead to feelings of resentment, helplessness, and loss of self-esteem.

Aggressive communicators, on the other hand, express their feelings and opinions at the expense of others'. They place their personal rights above others', failing to respect other person's perspectives, needs or feelings.

In contrast, assertive communication respects the rights and needs of all involved parties. It stands at the healthy balance point between passive and aggressive communication. Assertive communicators express their ideas openly and honestly, without violating the rights of others.

2.4. Elements of Assertive Communication

Assertive communication is more than just the words we use. It involves one's body language, tone, and overall attitude. Let's dissect the different aspects of assertive communication:

1. *Clarity*: Clear messages eliminate confusion. Be specific about your needs, wants and feelings. Avoid jargon and be concise when explaining your perspective.

2. *Honesty*: When you are honest about your emotions, it builds trust and maintains obviously authenticity.

3. *Open-Mindedness*: Assertive communication requires us to be receptive to feedback and open to other perspectives that may differ from ours.

4. *Body Language*: Non-verbal cues are as important as the words spoken. Effective assertive communication involves maintaining steady eye contact, open body postures, and an unwavering voice.

5. *Empathy*: Understand the feelings of others and express your understanding to others. It shows your respect for their perspective.

2.5. Communication Styles and Impact

Let's examine the four primary communication styles: passive, aggressive, passive-aggressive, and assertive, and their psychological impact.

Passive communicators often feel helpless, ignored, or overlooked. They'll likely experience low self-esteem and potential feelings of resentment.

Aggressive communicators may initially feel satisfied or powerful after an interaction. However, over time, the continual violation of others' rights and dismissing others' feelings may lead to isolation or hostility.

Passive-aggressive communicators often feel victimised and project their negative emotions indirectly, leading to a lack of trust and unstable relationships.

Assertive communicators, however, tend to feel empowered and respected. They often experience healthier relationships and greater self-confidence.

In conclusion, understanding and embracing assertive communication is pivotal to express oneself effectively, ensure mutual respect, maintain healthy relationships, and promote psychological wellness. With this foundation in place, you are ready to embark on mastering the different techniques to practice assertive communication. Your journey towards setting healthy boundaries and improving your overall life balance, awaits!

Chapter 3. Understanding Healthy Boundaries: What they are and Why they Matter?

Healthy boundaries serve as the invisible lines that define our individual personal space—both physical and emotional. They express the extent of our comfort and tolerance level with other's behaviors towards us, and vice versa, thus establishing clear guidelines about how we prefer to be treated by others. Without healthy boundaries, we become susceptible to fulfilling others' needs over our own, leading to stress, resentment, and loss of self.

3.1. Defining Healthy Boundaries

In its simplest form, a boundary is a limit defining you in relation to someone or to something. However, it's far from just a physical line that marks where your territory ends and someone else's begins. Boundaries are essential to healthy relationships and, really, a healthy life. Setting and sustaining boundaries allows us to maintain our self-identity, conserve emotional energy, and engage in positive self-care.

A situation wherein healthy boundaries are not maintained often results in emotional distress, enabling behavior, and stunted personal growth. Conversely, understanding and implementing firm yet respectful boundaries are key factors for psychological well-being, improved self-esteem, and enriched relationships.

3.2. The Importance of Healthy Boundaries

Healthy boundaries create a separation between our own feelings, needs, and expectations from those of others. This separation is critical for our mental and emotional health as it helps us maintain our individual identity, cultivate autonomy, and foster mutual respect in our relationships.

These boundaries define where we end, outlines what is our responsibility as well as where others' responsibilities start. This demarcation protects us from being overwhelmed by the problems of others, instead of allowing us to focus on our personal emotional and developmental needs.

Further, healthy boundaries lay the foundation of every relationship—personal, professional, or casual. By setting the parameters, they ensure that the relationship nurtures and supports our growth without infringing on our personal space, thus assisting us in forming authentic connections grounded in mutual respect and understanding.

3.3. Understanding Personal versus Professional Boundaries

While personal boundaries are the limits we set in personal relationships involving family, friends, partners, and acquaintances, professional boundaries are the limits we set in our workplace interactions. They ensure professionalism, respect, and fair treatment in all work-related situations.

Personal boundaries typically cover areas like physical touch, personal space, privacy, emotional boundaries, and sexual boundaries. In contrast, professional boundaries might discuss issues such as workload distribution, allocation of responsibilities, maintaining a respectful and non-threatening environment, and acknowledging the personal space and work style of others.

3.4. How to Identify If Your Boundaries Need Adjustment

Unhealthy boundaries are often characterized by feeling used, not valued, or uncomfortable in various relationships. They occur when we let others overstep, manipulate, or control us, leading to feelings of frustration, resentment, and disappointment.

Observe if you frequently feel overwhelmed by others' needs, or if you're frequently sacrificing your needs for others. These could signify that your boundaries need adjustment.

It is essential to reassess your boundaries periodically and make necessary adjustments to ensure you are not investing your time and energy into unhealthy or one-sided relationships. Reevaluating your boundaries also acts as an intensive personal growth exercise, forcing you to thoroughly understand your needs, values, and tolerances.

3.5. Setting Healthy Boundaries

The initial step in setting healthy boundaries is self-reflection. Understand what you value, what you need, and what makes you feel comfortable. Once you have this understanding, communicate these to the relevant people in your life.

This may involve uncomfortable conversations, but remember that your comfort and wellbeing is paramount. It's okay to say no and express your needs and feelings openly and honestly. It can be as simple as letting your friend know that you would prefer they not invite others when you have made plans to spend time together.

In conclusion, understanding and setting healthy boundaries are crucial for personal and professional life. They empower us to take control of our relationships and maintain our emotional health. By implementing these boundaries, we eliminate negativity, enhance our self-esteem, and cultivate healthier, more respectful relationships. So, let's start our journey towards establishing our personal boundaries today.

Chapter 4. Speak Up: Mastering the Art of Saying 'No'

Starting on a journey towards mastering the art of saying 'No' can be challenging, yet epoch-making. For too long, many individuals have suffered the crippling effects of dysfunctional communication, mostly stemming from an inability to affirmatively express dissent or disapproval. It's about time we change the narrative!

4.1. Root Causes for Difficulty in Saying 'No'

A majority of people find it challenging to say 'No' due to various reasons. They may fear conflict, rejection, or the possibility of seeming "uncaring." These fears are often tied to cultural norms and personal upbringing. Some individuals, especially those raised in environments where their needs and voices were overlooked or suppressed, carry the weight of this upbringing into their adult lives. Their internal narrative may equate saying 'No' to being 'selfish,' 'difficult,' or 'unliked,' causing them to overextend themselves in an attempt to please others. This practice, however, leads to burnout and resentment, both of which can severely impact a person's well-being and the quality of their relationships.

4.2. The Power of 'No'

Saying 'No' doesn't necessarily have to denote negativity. It is a powerful tool for preserving your mental and physical health, maintaining your integrity, and respecting your values. It creates space for you to focus on what's truly important and respect your boundaries.

1. *Freedom to Choose*: When you're capable of saying 'No,' you can freely engage in activities and relationships that align with your values and personal life goals.

2. *Self-Preservation*: Saying 'No' to requests that drain or cause undue stress helps prevent burnout and preserve one's physical health.

3. *Maintaining Integrity*: Upholding one's 'No' in the face of pressure nurtures self-respect and also earns the respect of others.

4. *Promoting Authenticity*: It fosters genuine relationships built on respect for individual boundaries and autonomy, not just compliance and people-pleasing.

4.3. Techniques for Saying 'No'

It's not enough simply to understand the power of 'No'; putting it into practice might be mysterious for many. Here are some comprehensive strategies to make this process easier:

1. *Use Clear and Firm Language*: Avoid using ambiguous terms that may lead the other party to think you'll change your mind. Firm yet respectful language will communicate your stance.

2. *Pre-emptive 'No'*: To circumvent uncomfortable situations, anticipate frequent or recurring requests that you're likely to refuse and address them beforehand.

3. *Delay Your Response*: If you're unsure, it's perfectly acceptable to ask for time to think over the request before giving an answer.

4. *Reiterate Your 'No'*: Some may continue to push after an initial 'No.' Keep reaffirming your response firmly and respectfully until the requester understands your stance.

4.4. Respectful Refusing: The 'No' Sandwich

Communication experts recommend the 'No' sandwich technique as an efficient method of refusing a request gracefully. The idea is to cushion the 'No' between two positive or neutral statements, reducing the potential negative impact of refusal. For example:

1. *First Layer: Positive or Neutral Affirmation*: "I understand why you've asked me, and I appreciate your confidence in me..."

2. *Middle Layer: The 'No' Statement*: "...but I'm unfortunately unable to help with that at the moment..."

3. *Final Layer: Positive or Neutral Conclusion*: "...I'm confident you'll find the right person for this task."

The 'No' sandwich is a way to say 'No' without being hurtful or making the requester feel devalued.

4.5. Assertive 'No' versus Aggressive 'No'

While asserting your 'No,' it's essential to strike a balance and avoid sliding into the realm of aggression. While assertiveness respects the rights of all parties involved, aggression can undermine the requester's feelings and needs.

1. *Assertive 'No'*: "I'm unable to take on this task as I have a lot on my plate currently."

2. *Aggressive 'No'*: "Why can't you do it yourself? I'm not your personal lackey."

Becoming proficient in saying 'No' can be a liberating, powerful, and transformative experience. It forms the backbone of assertive communication and is crucial for setting and maintaining healthy relationship boundaries. By understanding and employing the strategies discussed, you've taken a significant stride towards embracing your true potential and power. As the axiom goes, 'change begins at the end of your comfort zone,' and saying 'No' is often the first step.

Remember, the art of saying 'No' is a skill like any other that demands learning, practice, and time. Be patient with yourself on this enriching journey towards self-assertion and healthy boundary-setting. The future you will thank you for it!

Chapter 5. Assertiveness in Action: Real-life Case Studies

Assertiveness is more than just a communication style. It is about being aware of your rights while respecting those of others. It is often misunderstood and incorrectly associated with aggression, whereas it actually stands for balance, respect, and self-expression. Now, let's dive into some real-life case scenarios to better illustrate how assertiveness can be applied in various spheres of life.

5.1. Case Study 1: Office Conflicts

In a large multinational corporation, a project manager named Alice often felt overwhelmed by her colleague Bob's habit of delegating his tasks to her. Bob was senior to Alice but not her direct supervisor. He was positioning himself as a team player, but his behavior was adding extra, unsolicited work to Alice's already full plate.

After learning about assertive communication and recognizing her entitlement to healthy boundaries, Alice decided to address the issue. She arranged a meeting with Bob and laid out her concerns, "Bob, I value our cooperation and understand the mounting pressure we both face. However, I've noticed that you delegate tasks assigned to you to me frequently. This affects my own duties and decreases my productivity. Can we revisit our working model and ensure each of us is responsible for our tasks?"

By explaining her feelings and concerns without being passive or aggressive, Alice addressed the issue and prompted a conversation about tasks distribution within the team. Bob acknowledged his misstep and promised to review his work practices.

5.2. Case Study 2: Family Boundaries

In families, boundary setting can often become an issue, specifically when it comes to respecting personal space and time. Consider Sarah, a mother of two kids and a full-time professional.

As much as Sarah loved her family, she struggled with the absence of "me" time. After learning about assertive communication, she talked to her family, saying, "I treasure spending time with all of you, but it is equally crucial for me to have some personal time. I would appreciate an hour each day for my activities. During this time, I would not attend to routine matters. Is this something we can agree upon?"

By clearly stating her needs and being open for the discussion, Sarah successfully implemented new boundaries while maintaining family harmony.

5.3. Case Study 3: Friendships

Consider the case of David, whose friend Kevin would frequently cancel plans last-minute without respect for David's time. Previously, David would accept this behavior to avoid confrontation. Once he learned about assertive communication, David addressed the issue, "Kevin, when you cancel plans at the last minute, it communicates disregard for my time. Can we agree to inform each other well in advance if we cannot make it?"

David's assertive approach helped Kevin realize his behavior's impact. He apologized and promised to be more considerate in the future.

5.4. Case Study 4: Romantic Relationships

In romantic relationships, assertiveness plays a crucial role in maintaining balance and mutual respect. Lisa and Mike, a couple in a long-term relationship, faced difficulty maintaining independence due to Mike's insecurities.

Lisa worked late hours, which Mike resented. Instead of succumbing to the resentment or reacting aggressively, Lisa chose the assertive route. She explained, "Mike, I understand your concerns. However, my career is also crucial to me. It doesn't diminish my love for you. Can we discuss ways to reconcile working late with quality time together?"

Lisa's assertive approach opened a dialogue with Mike, enabling them to find compromises that preserved Lisa's independence and satisfied Mike's need for security.

These case studies highlight the power of assertive communication across various realms of life. Incorporating assertiveness enhances your respect for yourself and others, paving the path for harmony and a satisfying life balance.

Chapter 6. The Roadblocks: Overcoming Communication Obstacles

From a minimalist approach where one barely shares or expresses one's needs, to an aggressive approach where one bulldozes through others' boundaries, communication styles have a huge spectrum. As we begin to introspect, we'll identify the various roadblocks that often stymie effective communication, hampering our ability to assert our feelings and set healthier boundaries. These obstacles might be created by personal insecurities, societal pressures, or the fear of conflicts. Let's dissect each of these roadblocks first before presenting strategies to overcome them.

6.1. Fear of Rejection

One of the primary obstacles many of us face in being assertive is the fear of rejection. This fear often roots itself in our need for acceptance, for being a part of a community or group. We hesitate to voice our needs and set personal boundaries, worrying that doing so may cause us to be ostracized or at worst, result in conflict.

First, remember that everyone has a right to opinions and feelings. Asserting them doesn't make you less likable. Instead, it might help others respect you for your honesty. Always frame your requests or refusals in a non-threatening manner. The key lies in striking a balance between getting your point across without infringing upon others' boundaries.

6.2. Negative Self-Belief

Negative self-belief is another prominent roadblock. Perhaps you might think you're 'not good enough' or fear appearing 'selfish' or 'rude' while being assertive. Here, it's important to understand the distinction between assertiveness and aggressiveness. While the former resonates with respect for both parties involved, the latter tends to prioritize one's own needs over others.

You aren't being selfish by expressing your needs or setting boundaries. Instead, you are respecting your well-being and demonstrating self-love. Free yourself from the clutches of negative self-belief and indulge in self-reflection to get at the root of these beliefs. Counteract with positive affirmations to foster a more assertive self-image.

6.3. Lack of Clarity and Confidence

Unclear thoughts and lack of confidence often dampen our assertive communication. This can stem from not fully understanding what we want or need from a situation. Take time to reflect, get clear on what matters most to you, understand your limits, and start asserting them.

Building confidence, on the other hand, involves a commitment to self-improvement and the courage to tackle challenges head-on. Recognizing your self-worth and cultivating self-assurance might take practice, but remember, persistence is key. Start by making small assertive statements and gradually increase the stakes as your confidence grows.

6.4. Societal Pressure and Peer Influence

Societal standards and norms can heavily influence our behaviour. You might feel pressurized to conform, leading to suppression of your true feelings or needs. It is vital to realize that fulfilling others' expectations at the expense of your own comfort or peace is neither necessary nor sustainable.

To overcome this, acknowledge that it is okay not to partake in everything. Choose what resonates with your personal values and feel empowered for doing so. Understand that saying 'no' is not an offense, but a reinforcement of your personal boundaries.

6.5. Fear of Conflict

Anxiety about disagreements or confrontations frequently acts as a barrier to effective communication. It clouds judgment, stifles assertiveness, and breeds passive-aggressiveness. Remember, though conflicts are unpleasant, sometimes they pave the way for deeper understanding, better solutions, and healthier relationships.

A constructive way to voice your opinions without inciting conflict is to use 'I' statements. Instead of blaming the other person, express how their actions made you feel. This promotes empathy and reduces defensive reactions, thereby transforming potential arguments into meaningful dialogues.

6.6. Difficulty in Saying No

Saying no can be daunting. But not saying no, when you want to, can lead to resentment, stress, and burnout. It is important to realize that your time and resources are valuable, and you have the right to prioritize them as per your desires and needs.

Often, the fear of disappointing others stops us from saying no. Try to drum in the fact that you can't be everything for everyone. Assert your right to say no without feeling guilty. It's crucial to remember: a gentle 'no' is better than a resentful 'yes'.

As you navigate your personalized journey towards assertive

communication, keep these stumbling blocks and their solutions in mind. Overcoming these obstacles will not just help you assert your needs and set healthier boundaries, but will also assist you in becoming a more self-assured, respectful communicator. Remember, mastering assertiveness is not an overnight journey; it requires practice, perseverance, and patience.

Chapter 7. Building Emotional Intelligence for Assertive Dialogue

Understanding your emotions is the cornerstone to assertive dialogue. It paves the way to self-awareness, sympathy towards others, and effective communication. It's this proficiency that provides the clarity to distinguish your needs and craft constructive dialogues. Consequently, building Emotional intelligence is a vital cog in the wheel of assertive communication. Here's an exhaustive approach to equip with this ability.

7.1. Getting Acquainted with Emotional Intelligence

Emotional Intelligence (often abbreviated as EI or EQ - Emotional Quotient) pertains to an individual's ability to recognize, comprehend, manage, and reason with emotions. It's not only about managing our own emotions but also our ability to perceive others' emotions, respond to them appropriately, and interact effectively.

Dr. Daniel Goleman, a renowned psychologist, outlines five key components of EI: Self-awareness, Self-regulation, Motivation, Empathy, and Social Skills. Each component fosters assertiveness by fitting different pieces of the communication puzzle together.

7.2. Developing Self-Awareness

Self-awareness is your ability to accurately perceive your emotions in the moment and understand your tendencies across situations. It's about recognizing your emotional triggers and understanding their effects.

A solid self-awareness foundation allows you to express what you need confidently and openly, a vital step towards assertiveness.

Here are some recommendations to enhance self-awareness:

- Keep a Feelings Diary: Write down your emotions throughout the day and evaluate what provoked these feelings.

- Self-Reflect: Take a few moments every day to contemplate your emotions and behaviors.

- Seek Feedback: Regularly solicit feedback from family, friends, and co-workers about your emotional responses.

7.3. Applying Emotional Self-Regulation

Emotional regulation refers to your ability to manage your emotional reactions to experiences. Reacting impulsively driven by emotions may lead to sub-optimal outcomes. Emotional regulation is vital for stopping impulsive reactions and formulating thoughtful, assertive responses.

To enhance emotional self-regulation consider:

- Developing Clear Thought Processes: Try to rationalize your emotions. It helps to put things into perspective and results in a balanced assessment.

- Mindfulness: Meditation and deep-breathing exercises can help manage emotional arousal, providing a clearer headspace for assertive communication.

- Cognitive Behavioral Techniques: Reframe the negative cues in a way that they lose their impact on your emotions.

7.4. Focusing on Motivation

Your drive to achieve goals, regardless of the circumstances, defines motivation from an emotional intelligence perspective. Assertive communication requires this resolve to make your voice heard.

Raise motivation by setting challenging yet achievable goals, staying optimistic, and cultivating emotional resilience.

7.5. Nurturing Empathy

Empathy, another key EI component, compliments assertiveness by enabling you to consider others' emotions and perspectives. Empathy ensures assertiveness doesn't become aggressiveness.

To develop empathy, try to actively listen to others, embrace their perspectives, and respond thoughtfully.

7.6. Honing Social Skills

Lastly, social skills encompass effective communication, teamwork, and conflict management. These skills are critical for assertive dialogue.

Building better social skills can be achieved by practicing active listening, expressing yourself clearly, managing conflicts effectively, and co-operating with others.

7.7. Practicing Assertive Dialogue

Emotional intelligence forms the foundation for assertive dialogue, aiding in setting boundaries and ensuring constructive interactions. Assertive dialogue comprises open, direct, and balanced communication. Practice it by clearly stating your needs, expressing your feelings sincerely, respecting others' rights and needs, actively listening, and providing constructive feedback.

Adhering to these action steps will help boost your emotional intelligence, setting the stage for more effective, assertive dialogues. Remember, it's an ongoing process of learning and adapting. So, get started, stay patient, celebrate small victories, and build towards a more emotionally intelligent, assertive you. Soon, you'll see how healthier boundaries pave the way for happier relationships and a fulfilling life.

Chapter 8. Assertive Tools: Techniques and Tactics for Everyday Use

Assertive communication is not an innate skill. It is a learnable practice, that you can master using the right techniques, methods, and tools that have been scientifically proven to work. These are your keys to unlocking the beauty of assertive communication in everyday life!

8.1. Becoming Self-Aware

The first step in becoming more assertive is working towards understanding oneself. Self-awareness can bloom from two actions: introspection and feedback collection.

Interrogate your emotions and thoughts. How do you feel when someone overrides your boundaries? Do you tend to bite your tongue for fear of upsetting others, even at your own expense? Do you tend to suppress your own needs? Identify these patterns first.

Gather feedback from your peers, friends, and family. Do they think you're assertive? How do they perceive your responses in different situations? This external insight can be invaluable in revealing blind spots.

8.2. Express Your Feelings Tactfully

Vulnerability can become your strength. You can effectively express your emotions using 'I' statements. Avoid statements that sound blaming or accusing. Instead of saying, "You make me feel ignored," reclaim your power by saying, "I feel ignored when I am not given any (or enough) opportunity to share my viewpoint."

8.3. Using the DESC Script

DESC stands for Describe, Express, Specify, and Consequences. This is a useful framework for creating clear, assertive messages.

- **Describe:** Provide a factual account without judgment. For instance, "I noticed that the deadline for the project has been advanced."

- **Express:** Share your feelings about the situation using "I" statements, not "you" statements. e.g., "I feel overwhelmed because of the additional workload."

- **Specify:** Clearly communicate what you would prefer. For instance, "I would need an extension or additional resources to cater to the changes."

- **Consequences:** Convey the potential positive outcome if your request is met. For instance, "Providing either of these will ensure a quality outcome."

8.4. The Assertiveness Formula

Another tool is the Assertiveness Formula- it consists of 5 steps: "When you...I feel...because...I'd prefer...So can we...?"

This works well to diffuse confrontation while still asserting your needs.

8.5. Setting Boundaries

To set effective boundaries, articulate them plainly, unambiguously and ensure they're respected by steadfastly maintaining them. While there may be resistance initially, consistently keeping your boundaries will lead to respect and healthier relationships.

8.6. Saying No

Start by internally acknowledging that it's okay to say no. Communicate it clearly without feeling the need to over-explain yourself. An assertive "no" is respectful, concise, and firm.

8.7. Active Listening

Active listening is key in assertive communication. Not every conversation is about asserting needs; sometimes, it's equally essential to listen, understand, and validate the emotions of others proactively.

8.8. Open Body Language

Our non-verbal communication can often convey messages more strongly than verbal. Stand tall, maintain eye contact, and keep your presence welcoming, not intimidating. These subtle cues assert your confidence.

8.9. Practicing Assertiveness

Just like any other skill, assertiveness requires practice. Start with smaller concerns and gradually move to bigger ones. Utilize role play with a trusted individual to simulate situations and improve your confidence.

8.10. Dealing with Aggressive Communicators

Being assertive does not mean being aggressive. Should you encounter an aggressive communicator, maintain your calm, listen attentively, and respond assertively, sticking to your perspective without undermining theirs.

8.11. Navigating Passive-Aggressive Behavior

Identifying passive-aggressive behavior is crucial. Once identified, you can address it directly, expressing how it makes you feel and what you prefer instead, using the DESC or Assertiveness formula.

8.12. Maintaining Positive Relationships

Assertiveness is not about winning a battle, but nurturing relationships. Consistent respect for yourself and others, understanding, empathy, and kindness go a long way toward sustaining and enhancing relationships.

By mastering these tools and techniques, you can hone your assertiveness and build healthier boundaries, cultivating enriching relationships and achieving fulfilling experiences in your personal and professional life. Practice makes perfect: start today, stay committed, and see yourself transform into a confident, assertive communicator.

Chapter 9. Nurturing Relationships: Assertiveness in Friendship, Family, and Love

Assertiveness is a concept that everyone should aspire to grasp and incorporate into their daily interactions. While being assertive can initially seem daunting to many, it is a key communication skill that can boost your confidence and lead to healthier relationships in all facets of your life. From friendships and family dynamics to romantic ties, assertive communication can profoundly improve the quality and mutual respect within these relationships.

9.1. The World of Friendships

Friendships are among the most vital connections in our lives. However, they can also be a breeding ground for misunderstandings if not handled with thoughtful communication. It is here where assertiveness can step in to streamline your rapport.

Understanding your friends' standpoints and feelings, without mislaying your own, will serve to deepen the bond. Being assertive also means expressing your emotions honestly when a friend's actions impact you adversely, avoiding blame and prioritizing understanding. For instance, instead of saying, "You never include me in your plans," try saying, "I feel left out when I hear about outings after they have taken place."

Similarly, when a friend shares an issue with you, responding with empathy rather than solving the problem immediately can be beneficial. Saying, "I can see why you're upset" rather than "You need to do this..." acknowledges their feelings, fostering a mutually respectful environment.

9.2. Building Blocks of Family Dynamics

Family relationships often carry their unique complexities. Assertive communication within these relationships is critical, as it encourages balanced interaction where all voices are heard.

One method of fostering assertiveness within your family is through regular family meetings. During these sessions, express your feelings clearly but respectfully, and encourage other family members to do the same. By giving everyone a platform to voice their thoughts or concerns without fear of judgment or interruption, you minimize misunderstandings and make way for improved communication.

Additionally, assertiveness in the family involves setting and respecting boundaries. Suppose a family member consistently places unreasonable demands on your time or energy. In that case, it's important to communicate your limitations honestly - "I'm unable to take you to the mall this afternoon. I have prior commitments."

Respect is a two-way street that requires mutual understanding and consideration. And remember, while it's essential to respect the boundaries others have set, it's equally crucial that they respect yours.

9.3. The Dance of Love: Assertive Communication in Romantic Relationships

In romantic relationships, assertiveness plays a critical role in maintaining a healthy balance of power. It aids in avoiding resentment, setting boundaries, and fostering emotional transparency.

The cornerstone for assertiveness in romantic relationships is open, honest communication. This requires both divulging how you feel and actively listening when your partner does the same. For example, if a partner has done something that made you uncomfortable, instead of accusing, say, "When you did X, I felt Y. I would appreciate it if you..."

Setting boundaries is another crucial aspect of assertive communication in love. Everyone has different comfort levels, and being vocal about them helps prevent misunderstandings. It could be as simple as mentioning, "I need some alone time each day to recharge."

It's also worth noting that assertiveness in romantic relationships isn't just about resolving issues. Regularly voicing your love and appreciation for your partner can strengthen the bond you share.

9.4. The Power of "No" and Its Impact

The term "no" is short but exudes great power. It is a crucial element of assertive communication and boundary setting. Assertiveness allows you to understand and exercise the power of saying no without feeling guilty.

Many are conditioned to avoid saying no out of fear of coming across as rude or inconsiderate. However, constantly saying yes can lead to burnout, resentment, and a loss of self-respect. Remember, it's okay to prioritize your own mental and physical wellbeing, and sometimes that means refusing requests or invitations that you're unable to accommodate.

For instance, if a friend asks you to cater to a last-minute request when you're swamped, you could say, "I would love to help, but I'm currently overwhelmed with tasks. Could we revisit this at a later date?"

9.5. Assertive Communication: A Lifelong Journey

Developing assertiveness is an ongoing process, requiring conscious effort and practice. It starts from self-awareness and understanding of one's feelings, thoughts, needs, and desires. Make it a habit to express these with clarity and respect in your friendships, family, and love relationships.

Remember, assertiveness isn't about bulldozing over the needs and wishes of others. It's about maintaining a balance where everyone's thoughts and desires are equally respected. As you navigate through the complexities of these relationships, remember that every effort you put into fostering assertive communication skills brings you one step closer to more fulfilling relationships and a more authentic life. Keep practicing, keep learning, and keep growing!

Chapter 10. Professional Boundaries: Assertiveness at Work

Assertive communication in the workplace purposes to promote a healthy interaction that respects not only personal but also professional boundaries. This breed of communication is forthright, respectful, and designed to make your needs and wants clear without infringing upon the rights of your colleagues.

10.1. Understanding Assertions at Workplace

Assertiveness at work is about having your intentions, proposals, and points clearly verbalized and recognized. Assertive individuals are self-possessed and voice their views and ideas openly, candidly, and in a considerate manner. It's about taking the middle ground—not being overly aggressive to the point where others feel belittled or ignored, and not being too passive, where your ideas are barely voiced or considered.

In particular, professional boundaries indicate the lines differentiating one's work role from personal relationships and engagements. Understanding and respecting these boundaries ensures a healthier work environment and lesser chances of conflicts or misunderstandings.

10.2. The Importance of Assertiveness in Professional Settings

Assertiveness promotes efficiency by enabling concise, clear communications that do not leave room for ambiguity. This precision prevents miscommunication, promotes ease in decision making, and creates an overall formative environment.

Furthermore, assertiveness aids in reducing work-related stress by allowing individuals to express their feelings and thoughts without fear, thereby contributing to their overall work experience and job satisfaction. Assertiveness thus becomes a critical skill—deserving understanding, practice and improvement.

10.3. Keys to Assertiveness at Work

Being assertive does not come naturally to everyone, but it is something that can be learned, honed, and mastered.

- **Self-Awareness**: Understanding your feelings and emotions in different situations will help you tap into your style of reaction—whether it's passive, aggressive, passive-aggressive, or assertive.

- **Clear Communication**: Be direct, concise, and clear in your communication. Avoid any form of ambiguity that could lead to misunderstanding.

- **Confidence**: Believe in yourself and your abilities. Show faith in your decisions and stand by them. Respectful disagreement won't be perceived as argumentative if it is done in an assured, composed manner.

- **Respect others' rights**: Understand and respect the rights of others while asserting your own. Equal respect should be the foundation of all meaningful communication.

10.4. Setting Professional Boundaries

Clear professional boundaries not only protect you from potential burnout but also narrate a sense of respect for yourself and your peers. Here are particular steps towards setting professional boundaries:

- **Understand your limits**: Comprehend what you're comfortable with and what regulations are in place at your workplace. Understanding these boundaries will enable you to determine when the line is crossed and take appropriate action.

- **Communicate openly**: If a boundary is breached, communicate your concerns promptly and assertively. Delayed reactions might enable those behaviours.

- **Be consistent**: Once a boundary is set, uphold it. Inconsistency might provoke misunderstanding and unpredictable reactions.

- **Know when to seek help**: If a situation is escalating despite your efforts, involve a third party, usually your supervisor or HR department.

10.5. Assertive Responses to Common Workplace Scenarios

Let's look at a few examples on how to respond assertively to common workplace situations:

1. **Scenario**: A colleague consistently offloads their work to you. **Assertive response**: "I understand that you're overwhelmed. However, this is your responsibility, and I have my own workload

to manage."

2. **Scenario**: A team member is distracting you by talking overly about non-work-related topics. **Assertive response**: "I enjoy our chats, though right now, I have to concentrate on this task. Can we talk during lunch break instead?"

3. **Scenario**: You've been asked to stay late when you had previously informed about leaving early. **Assertive response** : "I understand the urgency, but as mentioned before, I have prior commitments today. I will be sure to prioritize this task first thing tomorrow morning."

10.6. Conclusion

Assertiveness paired with respect for professional boundaries is a potent combo for a balanced work-life and robust professional relationships. It isn't something to be perfected overnight instead it's an ongoing process. Understanding and practicing by taking small steps at a time can help you move towards assertiveness smoothly and eventually lead up to a wholesome professional persona that we all strive for. After all, being professionally assertive is about maintaining a healthy balance—between speaking up for yourself while respecting the rights of others.

Chapter 11. Sustaining Change: Long-term Strategies for Maintaining Healthy Boundaries

Change - it's unpredictable, challenging, and necessary. To sustain the benefits you've gleaned from assertive communication and maintain your healthy boundaries long-term, a comprehensive and strategic approach is required. The journey may not always be straightforward, but with determination, commitment, and the right tools, it is attainable.

11.1. The Backbone of Healthy Boundaries: Assertive Communication Considered

At the core of maintaining healthy boundaries is on-going communication. You cultivate assertiveness by continually practicing open, respectful, and mutual exchanges, thereby deepening your communication skills and bolstering your relationships. It is essential to consistently voice your needs and feelings confidently and empathetically, respecting others' perspectives without compromising your own.

11.2. Boundary Review: Adapting Boundaries to Life's Changing Landscape

Life's dynamic nature necessitates periodic reassessments of our established boundaries. Regular reviews make room for adjustments pertinent to evolving personal growth stages, shifting circumstances, or new relationships. Develop an intuitive feel for when your boundaries need revising and be ready to reflect, adapt and negotiate as necessary.

11.3. Reinforcement through Repetition: Practice Makes Perfect

The old adage is true – practice does make perfect. From acknowledging your feelings to stating your needs, repetitive practice helps solidify your assert and boundary-setting skills. It creates a psychological muscle memory, enabling you to respond assertively without constant mindful effort. By practicing regularly, assertive communication can soon become second nature.

11.4. Mindfulness and Emotional Intelligence: Nurturing Self-awareness

Mindfulness and emotional intelligence are key determinants of assertiveness. Cultivating awareness of your feelings, thoughts, reactions, and triggers is crucial to effectively understanding and managing interpersonal dynamics.

11.5. Building Resilience

Resistance or pushback can occur when you express your needs or begin to enforce your boundaries. Cultivating resilience is a vital strategy in handling such scenarios. Resilience cradles your assertiveness, providing enduring strength and courage to face oppositions healthily and productively.

11.6. Grounding Techniques

Grounding techniques can serve as anchors during challenging boundary-setting situations. By managing anxiety and improving your focus, these techniques help you maintain balance and reinforce your boundaries effectively.

11.7. The Power of 'No': The Ultimate Tool for Boundary Protection

The word 'No' is a simple, effective tool fundamental to boundary protection. While using this tool, delivering your message with confidence and reason, sans guilt or apology, is critical. The pivotal role of 'No' is undeniably significant in maintaining long-term assertiveness.

11.8. Continuous Self-improvement: Lifelong Learning and Growth

Assertiveness is not a fixed trait, but a learned behavior that enriches with time and continuous effort. Embrace lifelong learning and growth by seeking new knowledge, inviting constructive feedback, and staying open to changes.

11.9. The Role of Support Systems

Enlist the help of trusted individuals who understand your journey towards a more assertive lifestyle. Their support can be invaluable, providing space for fruitful discussions and honest feedback to help you maintain, adjust, and enforce your boundaries.

11.10. Celebrating Success: Acknowledge Progress

Appreciating progress, no matter how minor, is a key strategy to stay motivated. Revel in your successes, give yourself credit for every stride made, and remember how far you've come – it will fuel your drive to continue forging ahead.

Navigating this journey will require commitment, patience, and a great deal of courage. It may be challenging, but the rewards – self-confidence, improved relationships, and a balanced life – make it well worth the effort. Forge ahead into the future, knowing you're armed with the knowledge and strategies needed to sustain your assertiveness and maintain healthy boundaries forever.